While

In

Waiting

ISBN: 978-0-578-76102-2

Scripture quotations marked (NLT) are taken from the Holy
Bible, New Living Translation, copyright © 1996, 2004, 2015 by
Tyndall House Publishers, a division of Tyndall House Ministries,
Carol Stream, Illinois 60188. All rights reserved.

Scripture quotations marked TPT are from The Passion Transla-
tion®. Copyright © 2017, 2018 by Passion & Fire Ministries, Inc.
Used by permission. All rights reserved. ThePassionTranslation.-
com

Scripture quotations marked (NIV) are taken from the Holy
Bible, New International Version ®, NIV ®, Copyright © 1973,
1978, 1984, 2011 by Biblica, Inc. ™ Used by permission of Zonder-
van. All rights reserved worldwide. www.zondervan.com
The "NIV" and "New International Version" are trademarks regis-
tered in the United States Patent and Trademark Office by Biblica, Inc ™

Cover design: Visual Republic- Alexis Ward
Editing and format: Emily Bernhard
Headshot: Katie Robison- Katie Robinson Photography
www.katierobinsonphotography.com

While In Waiting

Our journey through heartache,

hope, and healing

by

Angela McCawley Lee

Table of Contents

This book is dedicated to my two best boys, Bryant and Lincoln. You two are my greatest gifts in life, and you continually fill my days with so much love, laughter and joy. I love you forever and always!

Introduction

It was November of 2016, and I was sitting outside on a porch swing at my cousin's house on Thanksgiving Day. While others were indulging in delicious turkey and all the fixings, I indulged in a roll and some pudding. That's all my body could handle. My morning sickness was robbing me of experiencing all the amazing holiday food. Even the smell of it made me sick to my stomach. It didn't matter all that much to me because it meant the little babe growing inside of me was healthy and strong.

I was talking with my Uncle Chris about everything I had been through up to that point, and he told me I should write a book. "You have a story others need to hear," He said. I chuckled and made some excuses as to why I couldn't do that. He dismissed all my excuses and told me why I should. He believed in me more than I believed in myself, and that sparked something in me. What he said kept running through my mind. I kept pushing it away and told myself why this wouldn't be a good idea.

A few other key people brought up the same thing over the course of the next year. They all said, "Angela, I believe the Lord wants you to write a book." A book is much too intricate to do, I thought. I will start with a blog. I constantly questioned if I could write a book. Would this be something people would want to read? There's no way my story is meant to reach a lot of people. I loved books since I was young. I always loved reading, and dreamed of one day writing my own, but I didn't think I was capable of it or that I would ever have anything to write about.

8

In April of 2019, I was at a retreat in Dallas, Texas. They told us to write one of our biggest dreams on a notecard. In no time, I wrote down that I wanted to be an author. I thought this would be my little secret. After everyone was finished writing, we had to go around the room and share what we wrote on our card with everyone. I thought, "Oh no. I never should have written this. Now, I'll have to speak this out loud and all these people will know." When my turn came, I said, "I'm nervous. I've never said this out loud, but I want to be an author."

That weekend in Dallas changed my life. I realized the only person holding me back from my biggest dream was myself. The next week, I started working on my book. Although it hasn't been easy at times, the Lord has led me every step of the way.

There were other dreams I had earlier in life that I went after and failed at, and I let that create a fear of failure in me. I don't want to be looking in the rear-view mirror one day wondering, what if? I want to look back and know I put my heart and soul into pursuing my dreams and let the Lord breathe life into the things He had for me. All I want is to follow what He has for me.

Thank you for picking up this book! I hope it speaks to you and shows you that you can shake off the limits you have put on yourself. Our God is still in the miracle working business, and He wants you to take his hand and run after what He has for you.

1

The Beginning

I want to take you back to where it all began for us. Let me rewind time and walk you through our journey—a roller coaster ride of the deepest heartache and the Lord performing miracle after miracle for us. I was born and raised in Oklahoma City. My childhood years were full of so much love. I grew up in a Christian home with my parents and a brother four years older than me. My mom stayed home with us, and I knew when I got older, I wanted to be able to do the same for my children. I grew up taking dance from age four, and my parents never missed a performance. They were at every single performance throughout my dance career, into my late twenties and after as I dabbled in dancing for specials at church. It didn't matter how old I was, I always found myself scanning the crowd looking for them before I danced. If I couldn't spot them before the performance, I knew right where they were when it ended because my Dad had a specific whistle and wave. It may have embarrassed me in my younger years, but as I got older, my friends and I both looked for it at the end of each performance. My friends thought it was hysterical. I would always smile and realize just how lucky I was to have parents that not only supported me, but also supported my friends.

My passion for dance led me to become a dance instructor. I dove in deep and spent

17 years of my life teaching dance. Those years hold some of my favorite memories and biggest pieces of my heart.

My husband, Bryant, was born in Florence, South Carolina. He was raised in Kingstree, a sweet little historic small town where everyone knows each other. He grew up attending church every time the doors were open. He played sports and excelled in academics. He was an only child, but inherited four amazing siblings after his parents remarried. He felt a stirring in his heart to pursue ministry and connected with a church in Greenville, South Carolina as an intern. That ministry moved to plant a church, and he packed up his car and moved from his small town to the big city of Oklahoma City to continue interning. He moved to a place he had never set foot and didn't know anything about. I am a creature of habit and love staying in my comfort zone, so I commend him for doing something so bold. Little did he know, he would meet the woman he would marry and spend much more than the few years he had planned in Oklahoma.

In 2007, I met a sweet, outgoing, funny and dapperly dressed southern boy. He always had on a sweet smile and a perfectly tied bow tie. We became dear friends because of our similar personalities. I think he wanted to be my friend because I laughed at all his less than humorous jokes. After a few years, our friendship blossomed into a romance with a few twists and turns, and the rest is history. On August 5, 2011, I walked down the aisle of the cutest little castle wedding venue in the sweltering heat and married the man of my dreams. I knew he was exactly who God had for me, and our life would be full of adventures together.

Once we had been married for a little over a year, we began talking about starting our family. I absolutely adore children. I devoted my career to children as a nanny and a dance teacher, but my ultimate dream was to be a mother to my own children. When I look back on my childhood, I always wanted to be a few things when I grew up—a ballerina, a dolphin trainer, an ice skater and a mom. Everything changed except my desire to be a mom. I remember writing about it in my school papers, and I toted around baby dolls probably far too late in life. I loved having something to dress up and take care of, and I knew when I grew up, I wanted a baby to call my own. What I didn't know is that when my life and heart were ready for the very thing I had dreamt of, it would take years to get there. My arms remained empty for many years, when I imagined them full of babies.

I vividly remember the conversation I had with my husband when we decided to start trying. I told him most people can take up to six months or more to get the birth control out of their system. All the women in my family had gotten pregnant relatively quickly, so I didn't worry I would be any different. I was constantly calculating when the due date would be if I got pregnant that month, and how old I would be for certain milestones in their life. I had it all planned out, as I'm sure many of us have. I had a picture-perfect life envisioned of when I would get pregnant, how old I would be, how many kids we would have and the exact layout of our cute little house with a white picket fence. The road ahead had a much different timeline.

I went off my birth control and we began trying for a baby. Days turned into months, and months into years. The comments and un-

solicited advice started when people noticed
most of my married friends were having babies
and I wasn't.

Why don't you have kids like the rest of your
friends?
Is there something wrong with you?
I don't know what's taking you so long.
I try once and I'm pregnant.
It's not that hard.
You are so lucky to not have kids.
Your life is perfect.
You're getting older, shouldn't you be starting
a family by now?

These are a few of the hurtful state-
ments I heard during the lowest point in my in
life. I don't write this for you to feel sorry for
me, but to realize the things we may think are
funny can be a source of pain. Be mindful of

the things you say to people. After many failed pregnancy tests and a lot of heartache, we decided it was time to see a specialist to get to the bottom of why I was unable to conceive. I didn't even know where to start. My normal OBGYN assured me I was young and had plenty of time, which I understood. At this point, we had been trying for multiple years with no pregnancies, so I knew it was time to seek a second opinion.

I prayed the Lord would help me know where to begin. There were tons of options on Google, and it was overwhelming. I logged onto Facebook that day and saw a post from a friend that I had gone on a missions trip with to South Africa. She was sharing about the wonderful fertility doctor she had gone to, and how she was now expecting a baby. I knew that was my answer. I reached out to her, and she was so kind and gracious to share her ex-

perience with me and give me all the informa-
tion I needed to feel confident moving forward.
I called to schedule a consultation with the
doctor, and there was a six month wait to get
in. While we waited for the consultation, I had a
small surgery we were told could increase our
chances of conceiving.

We went into our first appointment with a
positive attitude, knowing things were probably an easy fix. We met with an absolutely incredible specialist. He went over all the ins and
outs of infertility and gave us our first method
to get to the bottom of things. We left extremely overwhelmed and decided to take the
next six months to pray and decide how we
wanted to move forward. If we used a doctor
to help us move forward in having a child,
would that mean our faith in God was not
strong enough? The answer is NO! If I'm
putting all my faith and trust only in the doc-

tor, that's a completely different story. I wish I could say I knew then what I know now, but I would be lying.

This approach isn't for everyone. This is the direction we felt the Lord was leading us during this time. We were continuing to pursue the Lord and walk in the path He was paving for us. We prayed, worshipped, dug deeply into studying the Word, sat still, listened in His presence and rested.

The Lord kept telling me to rest. Rest my child. Let me envelop you in my arms and rest in my presence. With all the decisions coming up and so many options available, I felt like rest was a foreign concept. How could I rest when I was still balancing my job, teaching dance, being a wife, keeping my house clean and trying to have a healthy prayer life? My husband stayed extremely busy with his job in real estate. In the world we live in, people understand the constant hustle and bustle more than they do the concept of rest, whether that be physically, mentally or spiritually. We feel a constant need to keep going, and consequently, complain about being tired. Trust me, I'm speaking to myself in this too.

We need to find time to not only connect with the Father, but also to listen. What is He saying to you? What is the Lord working on in your heart? What has He been speaking to you? Don't be afraid to ask your spouse the same questions. If I'm not taking time to pray and listen, I may not know the answer to those questions. The Lord kept speaking this scripture to me—

"Come to me, all you who are weary and burdened, and I will give you rest." Matthew 11:28-30 NLT. This is still a verse I go back to often. The Passion translation says—"Are you weary, carrying a heavy burden? Then come to me. I will refresh your life, for I am your oasis." An oasis is a fertile spot in a desert where water is found. I wanted the Lord to be my oasis, but I had to let Him be. I wanted to drink deeply of all He had for me and let His love and rest wash over me.

2

Our Miracle

We knew the decision was a heavy one, and we wanted to make sure we weren't trying to pave our own road. We knew we could try to make this work on our own, but we also knew the Lord's promises over our lives. That's what we wanted. We wanted to walk down the road the Lord had for us in this exact moment. I was trying to go around the mountain in front of me and walk through it the way I wanted to— the way I built it up in my mind that it was supposed to go—instead of letting the Lord lead me through. It came to a point of complete trust. Letting go of everything I put my hopes and dreams in. Did I truly trust Him? I came to a crossroads and this was it. I had to throw my hands up. I can't do this on my own any longer. The only way I can make it through this is with the Lord leading me. I don't want the plan I made up in my mind. I want what He has made for me. My plans aren't better than His plans. The way I see this going may be easier in my mind, but what He has planned is the way I want to put one foot in front of the other and walk through it. I don't want to walk through it alone like I would be in my plan. I'm walking through it with the Father taking my hand and walking this journey with me, never leaving my side because He never leaves me. These doctors were given the ability to learn amazing things and procedures to help people struggling with infertility. We never imagined in a million years we would be one of the couples seeking medical advice and help having a baby.

After a lot of prayer, we knew it was time for us to move forward. This was the direction the Lord was leading us in. It was unknown and scary, but we knew we served a mighty maker. We went through a lot of testing, ultrasounds, scans and blood work. After the final round of tests, we would get a phone call with our results and the best plan of action to move forward and start building our family.

I will never forget the day we got the call from my sweet nurse. My heart was racing when I saw the call I had been waiting for come across my phone. When I answered, I had a sinking feeling, and we received devastating news. After reviewing all the test results, we had a 1% chance of conceiving children naturally. I calmly asked what our options were, and they proceeded to tell me it depends on how aggressively we wanted to proceed. We could pay tens of thousands of dollars to see more specialists and try a few different procedures, or we could do in-vitro fertilization. Of course, my first question was, how much does that cost? The total initial cost was equivalent to a new mid-sized car. That did not include initial ultrasounds or some of the medicines our insurance offered no coverage for. Anything that was associated with infertility or a specialist was not covered by our insurance. My heart sunk, but in that moment, I knew we would do whatever we had to do to raise the money and fulfill our dream of becoming parents. We knew the mountains in front of us could be moved with the help of our Father.

I hung up the phone and called my husband to break the news to him. To say we were devastated would be an understatement. I remained positive with him on the phone, saying I knew everything would work out. We will get the money somehow, but I wasn't even sure if I believed the words I was speaking. The things I was encouraging him with I knew my broken heart needed to hear as well. I wish I could say I didn't doubt things at that point, but I was hurting more than I ever had. Why? Why me? Why us? What had we done to deserve this? Why would we have to experience this when I had devoted my life to children? In these moments, I questioned everything. I questioned God and why He would let something like this happen to us. I hurt so badly, I put the blame on God. In that moment, I felt myself starting to question my faith. Processing deep and painful emotions is incredibly hard. Even though we were hurting, we knew we had a choice to believe the lies the enemy was feeding us or lean into the comfort and peace of our loving Father. Why was I putting the blame on God when He clearly did not do this to me? He wasn't punishing me for something even though the enemy tried to constantly feed me those lies.

God is not a God of 1%, He is a God of 100%. These are the words my Mom spoke to me when I told her the news. The statement stuck with me, and I constantly repeated it throughout my journey. I was putting every bit of my being into the percentage the doctors told us. I was letting my diagnosis and the in-fertility take over, weigh me down and define me. These are things I had an incredibly hard time understanding and processing through. I didn't know anyone else who had been through this before, so I spent the journey feeling isolated, embarrassed, ashamed and hurt. Many times, I wished I had someone who could say I know exactly how you are feeling. I didn't.

At this point, we had to make the decision to move forward and know this wasn't the end for us. We had to hold onto our dream and the promise of becoming parents. We didn't know how or when we would come up with the money, but we knew we served a big God. We began praying for a miracle in any way God saw fit. In these moments, our faith was pushed to the limit. Did we really believe a miracle could happen? Yes, more than ever. We signed up for the IVF class every couple had to go through to understand the process and expenses. Two weeks later, we were set to attend our first class with eight other couples. We chose to keep this journey private, sharing only with our parents and a few close friends we knew would bind together as our prayer and support team.

The day of the class, I was so nervous. I didn't know how we would raise the money to pay for the procedure. We decided to step out in faith and attend the class. My husband called me and told me to meet him in the parking garage because he had to talk to me before we went into class. I was so scared he thought we should change our minds. I told him I wasn't in the mood for surprises because my nerves were shot, but he insisted I meet up with him. I impatiently waited on him to arrive and noticed as soon as I saw him that he was overcome with emotion. I was trying to figure out what that meant for us. He walked up to me and handed me a folded-up check. I opened it up and saw a check written to us for the exact amount of our IVF procedure. I looked at my husband and said, is this check real? I was in complete shock and disbelief. I could never have imagined in a million years

30

the exact scenario that played out that day. That was a huge step forward in having our dreams fulfilled. I still get tears in my eyes every time I think of that moment. We received our miracle! We walked into our IVF class that day with every penny of our procedure paid for.

In Genesis 22:1-14 (NLT,) it says this: Some time later God tested Abraham. He said to him, "Abraham!" "Here I am," he replied. Then God said, "Take your son, your only son, whom you love—Isaac—and go to the region of Moriah. Sacrifice him there as a burnt offering on a mountain I will show you." Early the next morning Abraham got up and loaded his donkey. He took with him two of his servants and his son Isaac. When he had cut enough wood for the burnt offering, he set out for the place God had told him about. On the third day Abraham looked up and saw the place in

the distance. He said to his servants, "Stay
here with the donkey while I and the boy go
over there. We will worship and then we will
come back to you." Abraham took the wood
for the burnt offering and placed it on his son
Isaac, and he himself carried the fire and the
knife. As the two of them went on together,
Isaac spoke up and said to his father Abraham, "Father?" "Yes, my son?" Abraham
replied. "The fire and wood are here," Isaac
said, "but where is the lamb for the burnt offering?" Abraham answered, "God himself will
provide the lamb for the burnt offering, my
son." And the two of them went on together.
When they reached the place God had told
him about, Abraham built an altar there and
arranged the wood on it. He bound his son
Isaac and laid him on the altar, on top of the
wood. Then he reached out his hand and took
the knife to slay his son. But the angel of the

Lord called out to him from heaven, "Abraham! Abraham!" "Here I am," he replied. "Do not lay a hand on the boy," he said. "Do not do anything to him. Now I know that you fear God, because you have not withheld from me your son, your only son." Abraham looked up and there in a thicket he saw a ram behind him caught by its horns. He went over and took the ram and sacrificed it as a burnt offering instead of his son. So Abraham called that place The Lord Will Provide. And to this day it is said, "On the mountain of the Lord it will be provided."

A ram represents protection and sacrifice. Just like when Abraham was going up the mountain and was uncertain of how God would provide, we felt a similar uncertainty. The amazing thing is, the curve of a ram's horn is designed to not get caught in a bush or thicket. For the ram to be there and be caught in the thicket on the mountain was extremely out of the ordinary. It was clearly a miracle ordained by the Lord for Abraham.

No matter what season of life we are in, we can experience a waiting period. Whether it's waiting for a child, a spouse, a promotion, a financial breakthrough or an answered prayer, we must cling to the One who can give us peace and comfort. Keep taking steps forward. The Lord knows your heart. He hears your cries and your prayers, and He sees your sacrifices.

3

So It Begins

There's nothing that makes the reality of it all hit you more than a giant box of medicine and needles arriving on your doorstep. We were one week out, so instead of wallowing the week away, we planned accordingly. We were leaving on a plane to New York City for what we called our pre-IVF babymoon. Being the huge theatre nerd I am, I had always dreamed of going to NYC. I was all about the hustle and bustle, bright lights and singing and dancing. My husband pulled out all the stops for me.

He endured four Broadway shows! We saw my absolute favorite shows, Aladdin and Wicked. The costumes, singing, perfectly choreographed tap number and show-stopping vocals had me moving in my seat, reliving my young dance days in my head. Other highlights of the trip were the behind the scenes Disney Broadway tour, Wall Street and Top of the Rock! If you do the behind the scenes tour, you get to go in the archive room, try on costumes and play with props from the actual Broadway shows. My husband and I were the only adults on the tour without children in tow. In the end, my husband felt like he had a child with him because I was living my best life in there sitting in Ariel's bathtub. A redhead's dream come true! The skyline view at Top of the Rock was absolutely amazing. You could see so much of the city in a new way. Wall Street had me huffing and puffing by the end.

When our tour guide said don't doddle, he wasn't kidding! I couldn't have asked for a better trip.

On the plane ride home, the nerves started to hit me. I knew the process that would start the next day. The first part of injections happened at 8pm each night. When that time came, I started to panic. I asked myself, "Do you really know what you're doing?" I wasn't a nurse. Why in the world would they think I was qualified to do this? I wondered what I had gotten myself into. I didn't like needles, but I was willing to lay that aside, knowing what the end result could be. My husband hated them. Even the sight of them made him cringe. He did not want to be in the room to see it but said if I needed any help, to call him. I barely pricked myself and said, "I can't do this. I don't want to do this!" My sweet husband came to my rescue. He said, "You can and will do this. Remember what the end result will be. We are going to count to three, and on three, you are going to take the whole shot." One. Two. Three. I did it! I took the whole shot, looked up at him and said, "Oh, that wasn't so bad!" I had led myself to believe it would be much worse than it was. I think there are many times in life we work up a situation to be bigger than it is. Sometimes, all we need to do is take that step of faith or take that little push from someone who is helping us move in the right direction.

There were many times my knight in shining armor had to come to my rescue, help calm my nerves and remind me not to get so worked up about things. I had a good little system set up where my medicines were in order to make things go as smoothly as possible. I was cleaning one day, getting ready for some guests to come and had moved things around a little bit.

I remember my husband walking into the bathroom to me having a full-on breakdown. I was
crying and tearing through our bathroom. I
was in a full-blown panic because I thought I
had thrown away a brand-new bottle of medicine. I ran outside to check the trash and they
had already come and taken it away. I started
bawling right in the middle of my driveway. I
was crying, telling him how I would mess everything up if I couldn't find this vial of medicine
for my shots. My fertility clinic didn't have this
medicine readily available in stock, and this
was my last dose of it. I went on and on about
how I would ruin everything. My emotions were
on a much higher level than I should have ever
let them travel to. I was letting them take over
everything. My husband helped me calm down
and retrace my steps. It turns out I had not
thrown away the precious vial of medicine for
my last set of injections, I had only moved it

when I was cleaning. I put it in a safe spot where I wouldn't forget where it was. My panic set in and made me forget everything.

The whole process was proving to not only be hard on my body, but also on my mind. One of the things that helped me and Bryant the most was praying separately and together and staying deeply rooted in scripture. One of the scriptures I clung to was Jeremiah 29:11 (NIV)—"For I know the plans I have for you, declares the Lord, plans to prosper you and not to harm you, plans to give you hope and a future." Something beautiful and personal the Lord taught me was to personalize this scripture to our journey. This has come full circle for me, as we teach this regularly in our Moms in the Making support groups. I would personalize it and say—"For I know the plans I have for Bryant and Angela," declares the Lord, "plans to prosper Bryant and Angela, and not to harm Bryant and Angela, plans to give Bryant and Angela hope and a future." Learning to personalize and pray scriptures over ourselves was a very powerful tool.

4

Angels Watching

I was so used to staring at the same view of the doctor's office. It was a normal routine for me to walk in, the receptionist know my name and for me to sit in what I deemed "my chair" in the waiting room. I had the same view, started to recognize the same people and wondered over time if anyone else in there was going through the same thing I was. Was there anyone else besides the people I had seen at my class that were walking the same unknown road we were? I felt so alone and sometimes forgotten. Today's appointment was a suppression check—checking levels and having ultrasounds to make sure everything was where it needed to be so the doctor could safely overstimulate my eggs. Everything looked incredible, and I was right on track. I passed my test! I felt a whirlwind of emotions leaving that appointment, knowing that if all went well, in the next 15 to 17 days, I could be pregnant! I kept expecting something to pop up that would throw us off track or become a major roadblock.

I had another great ultrasound a few days later and went back again on a Saturday morning. Everything was measuring ahead, and they told me it was time to take my trigger shot that night. I felt instantaneous joy. This could really be happening! My body was accepting everything like clockwork. My nurse said she could tell my body was ready and acting as though it was preparing to be pregnant. This was music to my ears.

As I was driving home, I began to pray and couldn't help but get overwhelmed at the goodness of God. Even though there were still times I questioned why I was going through this process, I chose that day to know it was for a reason. I still believed through all the pain, tears and hurt, God was good. I kept seeing an image in my head of a beautiful blue color with a white feather. I knew I recognized it, but I couldn't figure out where from. A white feather is commonly known as the angel feather. It can be a sign of faith and protection. Blue is the color of the sky, so it immediately made me think of the heavens. I realized the picture in my mind looked just like the cover of one of my favorite books. The book is about different people's lives and circumstances, and how there are specific angels assigned to each individual for their mission. In that moment, I knew there were already angels in heaven praying on Bryant and I and our baby's behalf. I knew there would be angels surrounding the operating room, and I felt a sudden peace! I am not alone. Though I walked through days feeling so lonely because I had no one to relate to, I knew I wasn't alone. God always goes before me.

The infertility community is one of the most beautiful places. I have found so much healing, wisdom and community since going through my years of infertility. One of the biggest things I learned is that infertility is normal for many other couples too. I felt shame. I felt a lot of feelings that put me in dark places at times. I didn't know there were other couples out there struggling with these exact same things. I chose to keep this part of my life hidden. Looking back, I realize that doing that only caused me deeper pain. Now, I know this amazing community and all the beautiful people who are a part of it. There is so much help out there. Instead of hiding, we should look for resources, reach out to someone or join a support group. Many times, my friends and other people who knew me well could tell something was going on, but I didn't know how to verbalize what I was feeling. All I wanted was someone to relate to. There were very few friends I told what I was going through. I remember going to church on Wednesday nights and having to sneak out right before 8pm to take my injection. I always sat by the same friends at church because my husband usually worked or had showings on Wednesday nights. They started to realize every week around the same time, I got up and left and would be gone for a while. I had to mix up my shot and administer it to myself, and it took some time. One of my friends I sat next to each week would ask me if I was okay, and each time, I would say, I'm fine. I'm just having some stomach issues. That was the best thing I could think to say. I'm putting a shot in my stomach because of fertility issues, so condense the two and voila, it was stomach issues. The friends I sat next to every week caught on and knew something was going on. I have the worst poker face, so if my words don't tell you something is wrong, my face absolutely will. If my face's job was to hide my feelings, it would be fired on its first day.

The next week, I went to lunch with this friend and told her what was going on. It turned out the people she had nannied for walked the road of infertility as well and had to have IVF to start their family. They were blessed with beautiful twins. I went into that lunch extremely nervous, not sure how my friend would view me for what I was going through. I left that lunch having heard a beautiful testimony of a family being started through IVF and feeling refreshed and encouraged. I had never met anyone outside my IVF class that had gone through this before. Just knowing someone who knew someone that went through it was so helpful to me. I felt like that lunch was a God-wink moment for me. He was showing me I wasn't alone. That day showed me I needed to look for a community of people to surround myself with through this.

At one point, I thought God's will for my life was me going through infertility. I thought this must be God's will for me to walk this road so I can help other people. God didn't want me to be in the place I was. Why would I think that a beautiful and loving Father would want to inflict pain on me? I kept asking myself where I was putting my hope. At the end of the day, I want to stand on the truth of the Word of God. God wants me and my husband healed and not having to deal with this disease of infertility. I know His Word reigns true to this day. He is good. He fulfills his promises, and He knows the desires of our heart.

5

8:53am

A few weeks passed, and I already looked pregnant. I was so bloated from all my injections and medications. That evening, I took my last injection and trigger shot, and my husband and I took the time to pray over the week ahead. The next day was Egg Retrieval Day! The retrieval itself took about 45 minutes. I had nineteen eggs retrieved. We, along with our doctors and nurses, were very pleased! I was under good anesthetic and ended up saying some very loud things to

Bryant in the recovery room that I will save myself the embarrassment of telling you. There
were giggles behind the curtains from others in
recovery as well. I kept whispering things to
him—in what I thought was a whisper. It turns
out they juiced me up in the operating room so
well that I had no clue how loud I was actually
talking. When my sweet husband later reen-
acted what I was saying at the volume I said it
all, I thanked the good Lord in heaven I
wouldn't be seeing those people in the recovery room again. Cue the blushing cheeks!

My stomach injections were officially
over, and I pictured myself waving goodbye
and not looking back one bit. I was ready to
be done with them. As I was getting ready to
leave, they drew big purple smiley faces on
each side of my lower back for Bryant to be
able to see the exact spot my injections needed to go as we started them that evening.

Progesterone shots in my lower back were painful! The needle was so much bigger than the ones that went in my stomach. My husband learned how to administer them by my nurse, and he put aside his fear of needles to help me. He was such a champ! Sometimes our fears will face us head on and make us overcome them to help others!

Later that day, we got the call from our embryologist that ten embryos had survived and were continuing to grow. We were hoping to freeze a few after the transfer so we could expand our family more later on. Every other day we received a call with updates, and it made my heart so happy and thankful there was even the ability to do these types of procedures. What amazingly intricate work these people studied and performed to help our sweet babies grow.

Five days later, it was transfer day! On Saturday, August 20, 2016, we opted to do a five-day fresh transfer, with two beautiful little embryos. I was so naive walking into this day. I took some pain reliever an hour before like instructed and figured I would get the good stuff when I arrived. We decided ahead of time that Bryant would stay in the waiting room, and they would bring him to me once I was in recovery. I should have asked more questions. I had read many stories of people being awake, and some people being asleep. My doctor opted for awake, and I found that out the moment I was about to go back to the operating room. I quickly changed my mind and said I wanted my husband to come back with me.

I was a nervous wreck! Thankfully Bryant helped calm my nerves and made me laugh. Seeing him in scrubs, a mask and a hair net was hysterical. I'll never forget the moment I was sitting on the operating room table and the doctor came in to chat with me and get things started. He looked at me and said most of the time this doesn't work the first time, but we are going to try to get you a baby today. He didn't say that because he was negative or a bad person, but because it was protocol to let his patients know that. It was time for me to lay down, and I remember in that moment saying, I speak against that statement in the name of Jesus. I speak life.

Bryant was so incredible, sitting right beside me, keeping me calm and holding my hand. I was able to see everything and knew the exact moment the embryos were transferred. We were approved to use two embryos for the transfer because of my age, and the fact I had never had a pregnancy prior. The embryologist chose the two best quality ones for our transfer. The procedure was pretty uncomfortable at the beginning, (narrow pelvis probs) but the transfer itself, I didn't even feel. They told me the very minute the transfer was happening, and I took my eyes off the screen where I was watching everything happen and moved them to the clock. I saw the time was 8:53am. I knew in that moment, looking at the clock, this was going to be a significant moment marked in time for Bryant and me.

I was taken to recovery and had to lay with my legs up for an hour. I was discharged to go home and be on bed rest for 48 hours. The day after the transfer, we got a call from our embryologist for an update on the embryos left in the lab. It wasn't good news. She was so sweet and delivered the news with condolences and sweet encouraging words. None of our embryos were far enough along to be a

freezable grade. I was devastated! This meant
if this transfer didn't work, we would have to
start all the way back at square one and go
through the whole process over again. At the
time, I wasn't sure if that was something I wanted or could handle doing all over again. I was
on bedrest, so I thought about it on and off all
day. I remembered them telling me not to let
my body get stressed. I was trying my best to
rest. I chose to trust and let the Lord's peace
wash over me. I found myself begging and saying, Lord, please, if you do this for me, I will
never ask you for anything again. Looking
back, I realize how silly that was. I'm sure many
of us have been there before, desiring that
one specific prayer be answered. We are begging and bargaining with Him when He doesn't
need any of that. We don't get just one answered prayer in our lifetime. We see prayer

after prayer, miracle after miracle brought to fruition.

After my days of bedrest, I wanted to get out of the house, so I went on a walk around the neighborhood. I was tired of scrolling Pinterest and having Netflix marathons. When I got back home, I noticed I had some bleeding and was worried my biggest fear was coming true. I was worried I could be miscarrying those little embryos. After a call to my doctor, my mom and an encouraging friend, I climbed back into bed and tried to keep my mind at rest. I was told there were multiple things it could be, and they hoped it was just implantation bleeding. They reminded me to keep my stress level to a minimum, which I almost found laughable considering the circumstances.

I had to wait nine days after my transfer to go to the doctor, have my blood drawn and see if the procedure had worked. We agreed we would tell our family and friends who knew it would be a two-week wait from the day of the transfer to give ourselves time to process whatever happened, and hopefully be able to surprise them with an announcement. Those were the longest nine days ever! I was so ready to know if the procedure had worked. I decided to not test at home before my first blood draw. I almost caved a few times but decided to stick with it.

As you can gather, the next nine days, we were on pins and needles. We were on an emotional rollercoaster. My husband was feeling the burden of the wait and it was evident to his boss. She said something we clung to— God didn't bring you this far for it to fail.

I have never felt my nerves on the level they were that morning. Today was the day we would find out if the procedure worked. I went into the fertility clinic to have my blood drawn, and they told me they would call me in an hour with the results. That hour crawled by and came and went with no phone call. I sat outside of work knowing I had to go in soon, staring at my phone and wishing it would ring. An hour and forty-five minutes later, I begrudgingly gathered my things and headed up the walkway to the door to go into work. As I was walking in the door, my phone rang. I motioned to my boss I would be a few minutes, and I stepped back outside. Nervously, I answered to speak to my sweet nurse, Kimberley. Angela, I have your results and I wanted to be the first to congratulate you. You're pregnant! I squealed into the phone. Are you serious? Are you sure? It really said positive? Those were the sweetest and most exciting words I could have heard. I was hearing for the first time the words I longed to hear for almost five years. I felt like at any moment my mind would snap back into reality, and I would wake up from a dream. Almost five years of prayers, dreams, pain and frustration were being put to rest. Our little miracle was ready for us! I quickly hung up the phone and called Bryant to tell him we were going to be parents! We're having a baby! We prayed 1,643 days for our miracle, and God had answered!

6

Two Pink Lines

When I called Bryant, he picked up the phone and I yelled, "I'm pregnant!!! We are having a baby!" He said calmly, "Really? That's cool!" I was expecting a completely different response. I had built up in my mind this beautiful moment of me calling him, and he and I weeping and rejoicing over the phone. His voice literally showed no excitement at all. I said, "That's it? Are you not excited?" He said, "I'm in a work meeting right now, but I'll call you back." He was in a team meeting with all his coworkers, so he had to keep his cool because he had multiple faces looking at him as he answered that call. Looking back, it was a pretty funny moment!

After hanging up with him, I called my Mom. I had told her I was just going in for them to draw blood and check my levels. I was really hoping to be able to have some sort of element of surprise with my parents. I thought about that moment for so long. The onesie I would have made to announce to them, or the picture I would give to them saying the best parents get promoted to grandparents. It hurt my heart that we wouldn't be able to have those moments with our parents. She asked how things went and I said all my levels are looking good, and I'm pregnant! To say I shocked her was an understatement! I'll never forget her screaming into the phone and having to quickly hang up and call her best friend to tell her. I'm so glad I kept the day we were finding out a secret and that I got to surprise her after all. Not only were our dreams coming true, but so were our parents' dreams of becoming grandparents.

Telling our family and friends was such a fun experience. They were the people who stood by us, prayed for us and encouraged us through this whole process. I bought multiple pregnancy tests and took them over the next few days. I wanted to know what it felt like to see those two pink lines across the test after seeing so many negatives for so many years.

Walking into my fertility doctor's office for my first appointment since my positive test was exciting and nerve-wracking. Being pregnant was still surreal to me. I needed to see an ultrasound for things to really sink in. Once again, I played out in my head what this appointment would look like. I would go into my ultrasound and see my baby for the first time and emotions would overcome me. I expected to be a big messy puddle of tears. I was the opposite, which shocked me. I saw the teensy tiny baby on the ultrasound and at first, I felt nothing. Of course I couldn't stop smiling, but then I realized all the things that were playing in my head were based in fear. I was scared that after all these years of waiting, if I got attached to this sweet little baby, I could lose it.

Everything with our first ultrasound went great! Our little peanut looked healthy, and we were told my approximate due date was May 10, 2017. They only saw one baby which was a bit surprising to us since we implanted 2 embryos. This explained the bleeding I had after my transfer. I was fully expecting to be told that day we were having twins. In that moment, more thoughts from the enemy creeped in. Disappointment tried to attach itself to me,

but I wouldn't let it. I was over the moon happy
to see a healthy, tiny little baby! We would
continue progesterone injections, known as
PIO shots in the fertility world, until I was 10
weeks along. Then I would be released to my
normal doctor.

Once again, I built up in my mind that
since I had such a hard time getting pregnant,
my pregnancy would be a breeze. I was wrong!
The morning sickness started at six weeks,
and it came with a vengeance. If throwing up
was an Olympic sport, I was confident I would
take the gold in that category. It was worth it
knowing I was growing this tiny baby inside me
I had prayed many years for. I told myself I
would throw up all day everyday if I had to.
Little did I know, that comment was preparing
me for what was ahead during my pregnancy. I
would suggest not making that comment when
you are pregnant!

My husband went on a work trip to Mexico when I was about seven and a half weeks. I was committed to go with him, but that was during the time the Zika virus was very high, so my specialist strongly advised against me going. He said if I went against his wishes, I needed to stay inside and always wear long sleeves and pants all day every day. Can you imagine walking around Mexico with all of that on while pregnant? No thanks! I had to come up with an excuse as to why I changed my mind that he could tell his coworkers. The only people that knew I was pregnant at that time were his two bosses and their assistant. I wasn't ready to publicly tell people yet.

My mom came over for a few nights leading up to Bryant leaving to watch him administer my progesterone shots. By that time, Bryant had a great method of how we did things, and I didn't notice them as much anymore. I had become accustomed to it, and my skin seemed to toughen up over time. My mom was nervous, but extremely committed to doing them well. She literally practiced the injections on an orange leading up to giving me one for the first time. I could tell she was a bit nervous, but Bryant was going to talk her through all of it, and she had been watching how things went for the last three nights. We always counted to three so I would know when it was coming. We started to count, and I heard my husband say, "Mrs. Betty, it's not a dart." That is still hysterical to me to this day. My sweet Mom got so nervous that she started pulling her arm back and aiming like she was about to chunk a dart at a target. I mean, as long as it turns out to be a bullseye, it would get the job done! She ended up doing a great job administering them to me over the next few days. I'm so thankful my Mom was willing to step up and step out of her comfort zone to make sure things could still go smoothly while Bryant was gone.

When my husband was away on his trip, it ended up coming out that I was pregnant. I was nowhere near ready for people to know, so I didn't know for a long while that they found out. I totally get it was a little obvious. I'm terrible with excuses so I should have come up with a better one. I even saw all of them multiple times and had no clue they all knew I was pregnant. Looking back now, I think it's funny, but at the time, not so much. I would have loved to know they knew so I could have shared more with them. They are the exact kind of people you want in your corner.

I went to my fertility doctor every week until I hit the 10 week mark. My last appointment with my doctor was exciting and sad. I was excited because I was being released. I was so excited to no longer have to take injections daily. I was excited because that release meant my pregnancy was a strong and healthy one. I was sad because they had been there with me for so long through such a crazy journey. They saw me at some of my hardest and lowest moments in life. They saw me when I was hurting, and they were there encouraging me as my little embabies were implanted in my body. I exchanged hugs and many thanks that day with my doctor and my nurse, Beverly, and walked across the hall to the clinic to do the same with my fertility clinic nurses. They had become like friends to me. They knew me at my most vulnerable place, and I even knew some of theirs. To me, these people have one of the most important jobs! They answer their phones at all times to answer your questions throughout the process. They help people through extremely difficult circumstances and stand with them until their dreams become a reality. I am forever grateful for them!

We wanted to wait until we were 12 weeks along to publicly announce we were in fact going to be parents! We took the time before that to tell our family, close friends and coworkers the news. The reactions were absolutely priceless. Tears, hugs, screams and lots of celebrating took place. These people stood by us and prayed with us for many years. Not only did they see our prayers being answered, but they felt theirs were as well. Find those people! Find the ones who stand by your side, pray with you and rejoice with you! These are the people that stick with you through the good times and bad!

I had the sweetest friend, Brittani Purtle Photography, (If you are in the Oklahoma area, you must look her up!) do a photo shoot for us. It was so much fun! She captured a beautiful picture of some of my injections from our IVF cycle. I will treasure them forever! Not only did she do the photoshoot for us, but she also covered for me at my job for every appointment I had at my fertility clinic. I am forever grateful for her.

We announced publicly on October 26, 2016 with the picture on the cover of this book. We are changing our names to Mommy and Daddy. Baby Lee is due May 2017! "For this child I prayed, and the LORD has granted me my request which I asked of Him." 1 Samuel 1:27

11 days after our announcement was my birthday. That year, I knew I had everything I had been wishing and praying for. A few days after, I was extremely sick all day. I couldn't hold down any food or liquid. That was the level my morning sickness went to some days. I left work a little early to head home and get

some rest. When I was right around the corner from my work, a big Tahoe slammed on their brakes because the car in front of them did as well, which in turn made me have to do the same. My car stopped, but skid and slammed into the back of the Tahoe. My airbags deployed, and I immediately felt extreme pain in my stomach from where my seat belt locked. I was able to get out of my car and cross the street to sit down while we waited on the police to come. My phone was in my purse which dumped all over the floorboard, so one of the ladies involved in the wreck let me use her phone to call my husband and sat beside me while I cried. Thankfully, my husband worked right down the road and was able to get there in ten minutes. I was an absolute nervous wreck as I shared my side of the story with the police officer and other people involved. I was crying and shaking and just wanted to get to

the hospital to make sure the baby was alright.
I could already see bad bruising popping up
on my stomach. My car was hauled off, and
the guy said, we can't tell you this for sure yet,
but I'm positive your car is totaled.

I left the scene of the accident, and my
husband drove me to the nearest hospital. I
called my mom on the way and filled her in on
everything that happened. She was going to
meet us there. I walked in and saw her sitting
there with tears streaming down her face. I
know none of us voiced this, but we were all
worried about the little miracle baby growing
inside me. They took me right back since I was
pregnant, and I got all my vitals and blood
work. I was extremely dehydrated, so I got a
few bags of fluid. After what seemed like an
eternity, the ultrasound tech came and got me
and wheeled me through the hospital to the
ultrasound room. They squeezed the cold jelly

on my stomach and got the ultrasound started. Immediate relief flooded over me as I saw
my little babe moving all around. He was extremely active. I kid you not, at one point, he
turned his little head towards the screen and
waved, Hey Mama, Daddy and Grammy, as if
to say, "I'm just fine." I have my husband and
mom as my witnesses in this. Everything
checked out perfectly. He performed for us
the whole time, bouncing all around. It was absolutely incredible. I'm so thankful I was right
where I was in my pregnancy because my pelvis
completely protected him. If I would have been
farther along, it could have been a much different outcome. I'm thankful those same
guardian angels that were in the operating
room when our embryo was transferred were
surrounding my car, my baby and me.

7

The Celebration

We were so anxious to find out the gender of our baby. We had names picked out for both genders. Our boys' names were much more solid than our girl names, but we had one girl name we both really liked. Coming up with names and agreeing on them was quite the task. If you ever need some hilarious entertainment, check out a baby name book at the library or pick one up at the bookstore and read them out loud to each other. We laughed until we cried. We had one boy name we both fell in love with when we were dating, and I always imagined it being our first son's name. I had a very vivid dream of myself sitting in our nursery rocking a little boy and praying over him by name, Lincoln.

When I was 16 weeks pregnant, we paid extra to do a gender reveal ultrasound, because my doctor wasn't planning on doing one until I was 20 weeks along. As I'm sure you've gathered by now, patience is not my strong suit. My husband was going to be out of town on a work trip when I hit the 20-week mark. That morning, we were both so excited. We drove to the place, guessing the whole time. We went back and forth, and I changed my mind at the last minute. My guess was girl, and my husband's was a boy. We settled in and the ultrasound tech started looking. Of course, our little babe was being shy. I laid on my side, drank a coke and she tried for a good fifteen minutes before getting a few good pictures. The tech said, I don't like to guess, but I'm 98% sure it's a girl! There is a tiny bit of cord in the way, but I'm pretty positive. Come back in 2 weeks and check again, just to solidify that.

We cancelled our gender reveal party and moved it a few weeks later. I said I wouldn't hold her to her word, but the next day, my Mom and I went shopping for baby girl clothes and hair bows! We couldn't help ourselves. Have you seen how cute some of the baby girl clothes are?! My mother-in-law bought bows, hats and an adorable pink monogrammed blanket with her initials on it. I was already planning the perfect nursery with pinks, lace and a baby chandelier above the rocking chair. I couldn't wait to buy her all the princess dresses and sign her up for her first ballet class. I'm a dreamer and a planner. What's a girl like that to do? My husband stood firm by the fact he still thought it was a boy.

Two weeks later, we went back to the same ultrasound tech for our appointment. When I woke up that morning, I told Bryant I had a feeling it's actually a boy! Within ten seconds of our ultrasound, my feelings were confirmed. We were not having a little girl, but a sweet little boy! The tech apologized and insisted she was rarely wrong. We were thrilled either way for a healthy baby. Leaving the office, we knew the calls to our parents would be comical ones. We switched off calling our parents to tell them the news. All parties said, you're lying! That's not even funny. We sent the picture for proof! It was time to return some things and get into boy planning mode! My mind had been full of all the shades of pink, frills, hair bows and ballet classes. Now I needed to shift my mind to bowties, plaid and sports.

We had the sweetest gender reveal party thrown by my husband's work. We were having the first office baby and they were some of our biggest supporters on our journey. We already knew the gender, but it was so fun to reveal it to them with the cutest "Touchdowns or Tutus?" cake.

The next part of my pregnancy flew by. It felt like I blinked and week 20 to 32 was over. I stayed busy with nannying and teaching dance which helped time go by much faster. Week 32 came, and this day was a day I had been anticipating for years. After years and years of hosting and planning baby showers, it was finally my turn! My best friend and I went to get our hair done, and I chose to go back to a blow dry bar I had a tough experience at. This experience happened two and a half

weeks before we started our IVF cycle. I decided to treat myself to some relaxing time and
get my hair done at a blow dry bar. I sat in between two ladies. One just had a baby and was
spilling about the whole process of pregnancy
to birth. I thought, this is the last thing I want
to be hearing about right now. I can handle
this, I told myself. The girl on the other side of
me was talking about how she was almost thir-
ty and didn't have kids, and no one in their
right mind would push out a kid after age 32. I
was sitting in the chair next to her a few
months shy of 32 and still not pregnant. I
wasn't sure when I would be. She proceeded
to talk about her friend who had been through
many failed rounds of IVF and how sad and
expensive it is to have to do something like
that. She asked us, can you imagine how hard
it must be to struggle with infertility? Women's
bodies are created to grow babies. Those

poor women! I was sitting there a few weeks out from starting my first round of IVF.

In those moments, I wondered why my problems were brought up everywhere I went. I had a choice to make. Would I let these moments pull me down, or would I let them make me push even harder to get where I wanted to go? I didn't always make the right choice. Many times, I left places crying, but now I look back and see that those instances made me even stronger.

That day, I sat in the same place and in the same chair, with the same girl doing my hair, to redeem this less than enjoyable experience I had. I turned it into a positive, lasting memory. My best friend sat beside me, 28 weeks pregnant with a baby boy. That was something truly unexpected, and another sweet moment to add to my journey. I didn't know many other people who were pregnant at the same time as I was, and to have my best friend able to walk the same road at the same time was the absolute best. Our boys had a built-in bestie before they were even born!

My dear friends threw me the most gorgeous baby shower! I could not have asked for a better celebration. So many family and friends dear to me came to celebrate. I had friends drive in from out of town, and my best friend flew in from North Carolina. One of my dearest friends opened up her home, ordered the most gorgeous cake and had every detail planned so perfectly. One reason her hosting was so special to me was because she was the first person I ever opened up to about my infertility. I remember sitting in a restaurant in Breckenridge, Colorado, on a break during a work trip when she asked me if I wanted kids. She saw past my surface answers and could tell I was hurting. Opening up to her and having her hear my heart and share hers bonded us deeply. Anyone who has someone like Dana Drake in their life is an incredibly lucky person.

The rest of my pregnancy flew by. I was considered high risk my entire pregnancy, so I had my normal OB appointments and I went to a high-risk specialist for all of my ultrasounds. I also had to go in one to two times a week for non-stress tests. At 36 weeks, they released me from the specialist.

Since I hadn't been able to have a lot of family come to prior ultrasounds, we scheduled one last 3D ultrasound so I could have my parents and grandparents be a part of it. The baby was already sitting very low, so he was hiding a lot, but he gave us a few quick peeks of that sweet little face with the cutest nose and his sweet little plump lips. One of my grandparents had never seen an ultrasound before. Having my parents and grandparents there to experience that with me is a memory I will cherish forever. My Grandpa has since passed, so having these pictures with him there for such a big moment is so special to me.

8

The Birth

We had one false alarm three days prior to my scheduled induction. I will spare you the details as to why, but I'm thankful it did in fact end up being a false alarm because the nurse that checked me had a less then gentle approach to figuring out if I was in labor. I went back in early in the morning on May 8th to be induced. Since I was high risk and had thyroid issues and my OB was going out of town soon, induction was chosen as the best option for us. I was extremely nervous and had great anticipation as we were walked into the hospital as a family of two that morning. I knew the next time we walked out, we would be walking out as a family of three. This is the day we had been praying and dreaming of for so long, and it was finally here. For the past 4 weeks, I had been two centimeters dilated, so by this point I expected to be farther along. They got us all settled in our room, and then they got things started. The first thing they did was have my OB come and break my water. That was such a weird feeling. I was only 2 centimeters dilated when they started me on Pitocin which slowly started intensifying my contractions. I ended up having bad back labor, so after five hours, I opted to get an epidural. This part scared my husband quite a bit. He said the needle was huge, and I got electric shock in my leg when they did it, so I accidentally kicked him like a reflex. I was unaware this could make me shake really bad. These are the things I wish people would have told me ahead of time. I had my nurse come check on me because the shaking was so bad it was making my husband and mom a little nervous too. I progressed relatively well for the first few centimeters, but then I got stuck at a 6 for a very long time and ended up having to lay with a peanut ball between my legs for hours. First of all, I had no idea what in the world a peanut ball was. It was not very comfortable! Around 9pm, I was fully dilated to a 10, but the baby had disengaged. I tried pushing but he wouldn't budge out of his cozy little spot on my right side he was always balled up in. My doctor told me we would try again in a bit, and if nothing changed, I would have to have a C- section. I was super upset because I really didn't expect to need one. We even skipped over that part in our online birthing classes. Oh, the irony! I started running a low-grade fever, and the baby's heartbeat had moments of dropping a little, so at this point, a c-section was our best and safest option. They got me prepped and then had an emergency that had to be taken in the OR before me. I ended up having to sit and wait for an hour. That hour caused my nerves to really ramp up. My heart hurt because the conception hadn't gone the way I wanted it to, the pregnancy had been extremely rough and now the birth was going the exact opposite of my birth plan. I was letting my negative mindset strip away the fact that we were about to meet our little miracle boy we had been fervently praying for. I was letting circumstances steal my joy, and at the end of the day, all that mattered was that we were getting that sweet little baby there safe and sound. This is a moment I would fight for my joy.

I had a great support system of my husband and mom there during my 16 hours of labor. The anesthesiologist got me all set up, and I was taken back to the OR. As soon as I laid on that operating table, my nerves intensified even more. The medicine they gave me caused me to shake extremely bad, so I was terrified I would be moving too much and started to send myself into a panic attack. The anesthesiologist asked if I was alright. I shook my head yes and burst into tears! Are you scared? I shook my head yes even more. He yelled, bring me another bag of juice— she's freaking out. I now find that hilarious in hindsight! My husband grabbed my hand, told me to look at him as everything started, and he started speaking over me. You can do this. Your doctor does this all the time. You are going to be fine. Our baby is almost here. This is what we have been waiting for. You are strong.

You are okay. Deep breaths. I love you. I believe in you. I'm proud of you! As I'm sure you can gather, my love language is words of affirmation. He kept this up until I heard that first cry! Have I mentioned how much I love my husband? He was an absolute rock through all of this. From fertility treatments to the birth of our son!

My doctor held the tiniest baby up over the curtain for me to see, and then they whisked him away and Daddy followed. Cue the waterworks! My baby was here! I'm a mama! We are parents! My husband got to hold him and brought him over to me for skin to skin. He walked so slowly and carefully bringing him over which was so adorable. He wasn't super familiar with holding babies, so we had drawn up a whole plan of how I would hold Lincoln first so he could watch me and feel more comfortable, and then I would pass him to him. As you can tell, that plan became null and void because I was being stitched up while the baby was with Daddy and the nurses. Talk about beaming with pride seeing my greatest gift in life walking towards me holding our miracle boy. Cue the waterworks again! He helped hold him on me because I was feeling very out of it after the extra juice.

Lincoln McCawley Lee was born May 9, 2017 at 12:18am, weighing in at 6 pounds, 5 ounces, and measuring 19 inches long. After 1,896 days of praying for him, our precious gift from God was now in our arms!

9

The Aftermath

After I was taken out of recovery and back in my room, I started to feel a lot better, but I was starving. They told me I could try to eat some orange jello. Bryant called to let his parents know the baby had arrived, and I ate a little. I started waving my hands at him to tell him I needed a bag. I was going to throw up. He told me to hold on and he would get off the phone. He didn't understand I was about to throw up everywhere until I put my hand over my mouth. He forgot where the bags were

and quickly ran over with a cup. Yikes! I felt
way better after that. Turns out I wasn't ready
to eat after all. The first night in the hospital, I
was in a lot of pain. Bryant had to lift the baby
in and out of his bassinet for me the first few
days. Our stay ended up being three nights
and four days, and it felt like forever. Lincoln
had a pretty rough first few days adjusting to
life outside the womb and would only sleep if
he was being held. We had nurses in and out of
our room all night long checking on the baby
and me and bringing medicine.

I had the absolute sweetest daytime
nurse. She was checking me one day and said,
I have a very weird question, but did you use
to teach dance? I said yes and told her where.
It turns out she was one of my former dance
students I taught in my very young years of
teaching. What an odd coincidence. She really
got to know me on a whole new level. She was

now coaching and instructing me on things. Talk about a role reversal. I also had two lovely student nurses during the whole labor, delivery and aftermath. I always seemed to be asked if it would be alright if a student shadowed and learned with me. My doctor told me it was because I had a kind and caring personality and would actually be sweet to them. Some of them had less than exciting encounters with other patients, so I always tried to be as accommodating as possible. My daytime student nurse left her shift before my c-section, but early the next morning she got to sneak in and meet Lincoln. Her eyes lit up when I asked her if she wanted to hold him. You could tell she was absolutely meant to do just what she was doing. I knew she would be incredible when the time came for to be the one in control of the reigns. My night nurse student was the hilariously over-zealous type.

94

She very excitedly approached me and asked
if I minded if she was the one who removed my
catheter. The nurse said it was up to me. Her
eyes bulging in excitement and her big smile
told me I couldn't be the one to say no and
burst her bubble of excitement. I told her that
would be fine with me if the other nurse was
watching. She excitedly said this is the first
time someone ever let her do this. Oh my
word, what did I just agree to? She did so
great. I told her how amazing she was after the
fact, and how she would make a great nurse.
She beamed like I had just awarded her a million gold stars. It was quite adorable. Those
moments show a little compliment could go a
long way! She helped me with my first shower
which felt so incredible after not being able to
have one for a few days. I was finally starting
to feel a little better. My stomach was extremely sore. You never realize how much you

use certain muscles until you are supposed to be very careful using them.

We were all three sleeping great for the first time on our third and final night as the nurse came in at 2am and asked if my ice needed to be refreshed. Thanks for asking lady, but I'm trying to sleep. I know she meant well, but at the time I thought what I heard must have been a joke. My OB came in super early around 5am and asked how I was feeling. She said everything was looking great with me and my little baby and we could go home that day on strict restrictions, or we could stay one more night and be released the next morning. I was ready to bust out of that joint and get back to my own house to begin settling in as a family of three. That was still so surreal to me.

I had to be wheeled to my car, holding my teeny tiny little man that now weighed 5 pounds 14 ounces. He looked like a tiny doll in his giant infant car seat. He was incredible on his first car ride and held my finger the whole way home. When we arrived home, we only had a few hours to settle in and rest before the family arrived from out of town to stay for a few days and help us get settled in. I was on bed rest because of my c-section, so I wasn't allowed to do any lifting heavier than my little babe—no housework and no driving for two weeks. That was a tough pill for me swallow with how independent I am!

10

The Lesson

Becoming a mom was absolutely a dream come true. It was one of the most beautiful things I have ever experienced. It was something I prayed for and dreamed about for so long! Even still, I was so naïve to everything motherhood entailed. A lot of people sugar-coated things for me when I asked questions about being a mom. I thought there was something wrong with me because of certain feelings I had and different things I processed after having my baby. I was confident walking into motherhood because I helped other families raise their children for so many years. It gave me experience and prepared me for a few things, but everything is different when it's a child of your own. When I helped other families, I worked with kids to break tough habits and felt confident in doing this. It felt like helping families raise their kids was exactly what I was supposed to be doing. I was made to do this. The experience of having your own child is amazing and rewarding. I remember being so emotional. I would cry over every little thing. I was on a lot of medications because of my c-section. I cried every single day for weeks. I felt like I wasn't enough. I had a baby who had a horrible witching hour every night for two to three hours. I did everything in my capacity I knew to do. No matter what we did, he would scream and scream. He also would not sleep without being held overnight. It turned out he had a milk protein intolerance, so I needed to change my diet and start him on a probiotic. Those things were like a teeny tiny bottle of gold. The bottle was so little and cost $40. I probably would have been willing to pay way more because they did help. But no matter what we did, he would scream and scream. My husband headed back to work the week after Lincoln was born because of the demands of real estate and still needing to make an income for our family. Since Linc was waking so much at night to nurse, I took over all the night-time shifts. I was barely sleeping, and I was extremely exhausted.

Developing a new rhythm and routine is hard. At the end of the day, you were given the gift of being that baby's mom or dad, and you have to figure out what works best for you as parents. I had been given so much advice that it became extremely overwhelming. I didn't know the right thing to do. Some of the advice I asked for and some I did not. I had a few things set in stone I knew I wanted to follow, and luckily, I'm stubborn enough to not let that budge.

Everyone had a different opinion of what I needed to do. There were things I was very specific on because a lot of other things hadn't gone like I wanted them to. I really wanted to be able to breastfeed my baby. I was anti-bottle and anti-pacifier at first. I let some things people said make me feel guilty and make me feel like I wasn't a good mom. I tried a pacifier one time and then Linc wouldn't latch good at his next feeding, so they all got put away after that. He was such a champ at breastfeeding. He ate every two to three hours and would take up to an hour to eat, so by the time I was done feeding him, I only had a one to two-hour break before the next feeding. We had a beautiful breastfeeding journey that lasted a little too long for my liking, but I am very thankful for it. I am not taking away from it being a beautiful journey, just saying a mouthful of teeth hurt, if you know what I mean. Not only was I dealing with so many of my own emotions, I was also recovering from a major surgery and starting this journey of being a mom and balancing being a good wife. At first, I failed miserably.

Looking back, I realize how unnecessarily hard I was on myself. I let a lot of little things tear me up that never should have. Juggling it all was not easy for me. I lost myself trying to achieve a level of perfection I did not need to. In the meantime, I lost what mattered most to me. I was continually giving my husband the leftovers of an exhausted mom and baby that constantly needed to be held. I knew my husband deserved better than that. When you're trying to be the best you can be, you can let outside voices bring you down and become your inner voice. That is not a good thing. This goes for many areas of life, not only those pertaining to motherhood. It was not good for me. I put so much added pressure on myself. I needed to cut myself some slack because this was my first time doing this. I may have been other people's baby whisperer, but my own baby was not fazed by any of that whispering. Why did I expect myself to be perfect? I envisioned these moments so differently. We don't all easily fall into a rhythm right away, and that is okay.

You know those times you feel completely exhausted? I'm talking emotionally, mentally and physically. You feel super alone even though there are people constantly surrounding you. If you can imagine holding onto a rope by one tiny thread, that is exactly where I felt like I was. I was still holding on, but I wasn't sure how tight. At some points, I felt like I didn't have the energy to do anything else. No sleep, crazy meds and a baby with an insanely long witching hour every night pushed me to my limit. I couldn't imagine how people did this day in and day out. Those moments were more few and far between, but I knew I had to keep holding on. I had to know where my hope was anchored. I had to know to speak life into my situation. Truth be told, I felt like an awful mother. I felt like I had no idea what I was doing. Lincoln wouldn't sleep without being held, which was absolutely exhausting. I also struggled with post-partum anxiety. Every little thing would send me into a flood of panic. I literally felt like I was going crazy. I remember at one point, I was lying in bed one night when I burst into tears. My husband asked me what was wrong, and I told him I had no idea. I just want my happy wife back, he said. Some of you reading this may think, well, that was harsh, but for me, it was just what I needed to hear. I needed that truth. I needed to know that even he could tell something was off with me and it was time to take control. I needed to look right at that fear and command it to go. I needed to look right at myself in the mirror and tell myself you are a good mother. I needed to look at my husband and tell him I am and can still be a good wife. I was literally letting these fleeting thoughts and fears steal not only my joy, but my life.

For some people at this point, the best thing to do would be to seek help. For me, the Lord was having me travel a bit of a different road. I sought counsel from a few mom friends that struggled with this same thing, but at this point, prayer was my greatest weapon. The moments that it got too hard, my sweet husband would grab my hand and begin to speak words of affirmation to me, and then he would pray, declare and speak those truths over me. The stress my body was carrying felt so heavy at times, and I knew my baby could feel this. I knew I had to make a change.

If today you feel you are at that place, I want you to sit back and take a deep breath. If you feel you are at the end of your rope and barely hanging on by that tiny last thread, I want you to think of things in your life that are going right. There has to be at least one thing in your life right now that is going right. I want you to stop and thank God for that one good thing. I want you to thank Him and know that no matter where you are or how you are feeling right now, He hears you. He sees you. No matter what weight you feel like you are bearing today, He can take every single bit of that weight and lift it off you. He doesn't want us

to feel that weight. He doesn't want us to feel
like we have to carry our burdens alone. He
doesn't want us to feel alone. He wants us to
know He never leaves our side. He wants us to
rest in Him and let Him envelop us in His arms.
The Lord is my best friend and my shepherd.
I always have more than enough.
He offers a resting place for me in his
luxurious love.
His tracks take me to an oasis of peace, the
quiet brook of bliss.
That's where he restores and revives my life.
He opens before me pathways to God's
pleasure
and leads me along in his footsteps of
righteousness
so that I can bring honor to his name.
Lord, even when your path takes me through
the valley of deepest darkness,

fear will never conquer me, for you already
have!
You remain close to me and lead me through it
all the way.
Your authority is my strength and my peace.
The comfort of your love takes away my fear.
I'll never be lonely, for you are near.
You become my delicious feast
even when my enemies dare to fight.
You anoint me with the fragrance of your Holy
Spirit;
you give me all I can drink of you until my heart
overflows.
So why would I fear the future?
For your goodness and love pursue me all the
days of my life.
Then afterward, when my life is through,
I'll return to your glorious presence to be
forever with you!
Psalm 23:1-6, The Passion Translation

Now is the time for us to walk in victory.
Now is the time for us to proclaim the things we
want to see come to fruition in our lives. Let's
begin to speak these things into existence.
Let's begin to speak life and not death.

There is so much power in the words we
speak and the things we let come out of our
mouths. Let's seek hope. Let's take the negative thoughts we are thinking and find something positive to combat them. If you are sitting there today, looking in the mirror and saying things like, I am broken, I want you to take
a look back at yourself and say, I'm not broken. Look at yourself and see who the Lord
says you are. Speak the truth you need to
hear, and the truth you pour over others. Pour
that over yourself today, friend.

I am made whole.
I am the daughter of the king.

I am a son of the most high.

I am who God says I am.

I am chosen.

I am fearfully and wonderfully made.

I am victorious.

I am courageous.

I am a fighter.

I am strong.

I am a good mother.

I am a good father.

I am a good wife.

I am a good husband.

I am beautiful.

I am enough.

I am moving forward.

I am not my past.

I am not a mistake.

I am loved.

I am healed.

Take those things—those deep down hard things that you have made yourself think so much that they have almost become a reality. They have become what you think is truth. They have become what you think is normal. That is not normal. We want to speak life over ourselves.

If you had someone in your life who continually came and spoke negative things to you all the time, you would not want them to be a part of your life. They would not be healthy for you. Are your own words and your own mindset healthy for you? Are you speaking life or death into your situation? I want you to take a good, hard look at that today. If you are speaking death, today is your day to learn to begin to speak life. Even if its speaking scripture over yourself. Find scriptures you can hold on to and begin to speak those over yourself.

The statement everyone says to you when you first have a baby—it goes by so fast —is so true! Those first few weeks recovering from a c-section with lots of restrictions and the long sleepless nights made me think yeah, right! In hindsight, it absolutely flew by. I'm so thankful for my family, my parents, my amazing in-laws and my brother. They came and cleaned, cooked, did laundry, took out the trash and helped me and Bryant fall into a good rhythm of parenthood. Our friends brought meals, coffee and gifts and loved on our baby. Once Bryant had to go back to work and I was still recovering, my mom came every day. I cannot thank her enough for everything she did for me. She brought me my favorite drinks, treats and meals, and continu- ally encouraged me by telling me how good of a mom I was, even on the days I was being hard on myself. I learned a lot of lessons my first year of being a mom.

1. I thought I knew what tired was before, but boy was I wrong!

2. Stop being so hard on myself. Everything won't always get done, and that's okay!

3. Don't be afraid to ask for help.

4. It's a lot different and harder than I thought it would be.

5. I do things I never thought I would do. Sometimes everything you plan isn't what works best for your baby.

6. I never knew how much I could instantly fall in love with someone until I met my little boy. He's more than I ever dreamed.

7. He was worth the wait. As hard as it was, I would do it all over again.

8. Cherish every moment. Be in the moment. Take the extra cuddles and the extra time.

9. Breastfeeding is the hardest full-time job I've ever had. We made it fifteen months! If it's not for you, that's okay. Fed is best!

10. Take time for date nights and time for yourself as well! It's vital!

11

Woven

I remember the day I was sitting in my living room in Oklahoma City in my childhood home we purchased from my parents a few months prior. I was rocking my eight-week-old baby, so exhausted from recovering from a c-section and getting used to very small amounts of intermittent sleep. My husband said he needed to talk to me about something, and I knew in his tone it was something serious. Those words always make me nervous. Anyone else? I sat and listened as he asked me to pray about an opportunity to move to South Carolina. I cried because I always did when this subject was brought up. I told him I would pray, but in the back of my head, I knew I would tell him no because I always did. I didn't want to move and never felt like South Carolina was somewhere we would raise our family. I had told him multiple times I will never live in South Carolina. I could not picture my life or raising my son anywhere different than exactly where I already was. I love to live in my comfort zone.

We had just bought a new house, moved while I was pregnant and spent a lot of money putting together my Pinterest-perfect nursery, thanks to my amazing cousin who is an interior designer. This house was extremely sentimental to me because I grew up in it. We moved to the exact house I was rocking my baby in when I was just four years old, and we had created so many incredible memories there. I had it all planned in my head to do the same with my little family.

I began to take the time to really pray. I took the time to not only pray and ask the Lord what his will was for this situation, but also to listen. That was the key in this whole situation. Sometimes we pray about something, but we never take the time to actually be still and listen. We beg for an answer, but keep on talking, praying and pleading. I knew I needed a clear answer, and I remember clearly getting it. Every ounce of my being wanted to ignore the answer I heard or tell my husband I heard it differently.

I hated change. It made me a grouchy and grumpy lady. Would I let my fear of change get in the way of what the Lord had in store for my family? I knew if I looked back on this day and didn't agree to move, we could miss out on a lot of opportunities. I knew that day I had to say yes and take that leap of faith. I told my husband yes, I would move. He had the biggest look of shock on his face. He later admitted he never thought I would say yes.

I have had many hard days being away from Oklahoma. My family, my lifelong friends, a dance studio that holds a huge piece of my heart and a church that played a huge role in molding me into the person I am today are the things I miss most. Moving to a new place, where you know no one but your husband's family is challenging, especially if you are a relational person like I am. I adored my friends and lived a life full of visitors, phone calls, grocery shopping with friends, family within half an hour or less and so much joy. I loved my life and had put in a lot of blood, sweat and tears to build it into what it was. I didn't understand why now was the time, after all we had gone through. Was this the right timing? I had worked so hard to become who I was and get where I was in life. I have to throw all of that away and start over?

The move happened within two months of us making the decision, and it was extremely hard on me. I felt some very tough feelings to overcome and process. I kept looking in the rearview mirror of everything I left behind and looking to what I thought was a dead, empty road ahead. My parents helped us move and get everything settled, and then it was time for them to head back to Oklahoma. I lost it when I hugged my Mom. There I was, a grown woman in her thirties clinging to my mom, willing her not to leave. I had never lived away from my parents, so this was new territory to me.

After the move, it seemed like a desert season. I felt spiritually dry and lost. I prayed

over and over again that the Lord would help
me see things through his eyes. One sunny af-
ternoon, I was outside watching Lincoln play
as I sat in the rocking chair on my back porch.
Over the course of the week, I had watched
this same little spider build its web from our
back porch to the rose bushes on the other
side of the railing. Some spiders build new
webs every night, but this one continued to
repair the damaged places. Even when a tear
or damage came to it, it went back and re-
paired it again and kept on going. It kept going
even when it had a setback. The details were
so intricate. There were simple parts that were
done quickly, and other parts it spent days
on. The lines were seamless and perfectly woven together to make a beautiful design.
Those places took much more time, effort,
and patience.

This illustration made me think of our walk with Christ. There are parts of our journey that seem simple. We are happy. We are confident. Then a little tear, or in our case, a bump in the road comes along. We feel tested. Will this cause us to have a setback, or are we going to keep on going? Will we take the time to seek the Lord and repair, forgive, move on and keep pressing forward, or will this cause us to stumble?

The woven detail is just like our life. The web has detail, takes time and is intricately woven just like our journey. How amazing is it that He already knows every detail. Those tears or damage don't catch the Lord by surprise. He is our ever-present help in time of need. We don't have to continue to build our web alone because he already knows what the end product looks like. God is concerned about the intricate details of our daily lives, not just the big picture things we think about. It's the details that make a piece of art beautiful.

You even formed every bone in my body when you created me in the secret place, carefully, skillfully shaping me from nothing to something. You saw who you created me to be before I became me! Before I'd ever even seen the light of day, the number of days you planned for me were already recorded in your book.
Psalm 139:15-16, Passion Translation

Today I ask you, are you letting fear hold you back from something? Are you afraid of change like I was? It's not comfortable at all, but it's worth it to take that leap of faith. If you aren't ready to leap yet, just dip your toe in the water. I know you will and can get there!

12

Fully Free

While I was trying to figure out why I was here and what my purpose was, I started feeling a strong pull to be a part of women's journeys who were walking the same road I had. I saw that Moms in the Making was looking for new support group leaders, so I decided to take another leap of faith and apply to be a leader. It is hard for me to put myself out there or go for something I want without an extra little push, but this was something I felt strongly about pursuing. I went through the interview process and was accepted as a new leader. I felt like this was just another puzzle piece as to why I went to South Carolina. Sometimes what we are searching for can come in something as simple as a blog post or stumbling across an Instagram community you prayed for years you would find. It was right there the whole time.

One of the most important things I gained while walking the road of infertility was full healing, freedom and an incredible community from Moms in the Making. Some of the women from this group have become my closest friends. I know these are lifetime relationships. One pivotal moment for me was in 2018 when I attended the Moms in the Making conference. I went through my fertility journey so many years ago that I didn't even feel like others around me were going through what we went through at that time. We did the best we could, and I felt I had moved on from it. If I were being honest, deep down, I buried the shame I experienced from other people's comments as they questioned my journey to become a mom. I had a lot of disappointment, hurt, grief, discouragement and pain I buried so deep, I couldn't even feel it anymore. I planted pretty flowers to mask the rotten soil underneath so I could move on.

On the last night of the conference, they had individual prayer for everyone. They wanted to agree with us for our miracle. I already held my miracle, so I questioned if I should go down to receive, but a sweet friend encouraged me to go and let the Lord show me what He wanted me to pray about. I stood in line and prayed, and God revealed something to me. I didn't have much time to process it because I was close to the front, so by the time I got to who was praying for me, I had a hard time verbalizing what I was feeling. The Lord wanted me to grieve and let go of all disappointment—grieve the loss of so many of my little embabies that didn't make it. I let go of all my disappointment about the process I went through to get pregnant and it not going the way I had thought it would. I let go of the disappointment I put on myself of not being able to have it all together sometimes. I can be much too hard on myself. That is something I'm working on every day. I carried a heavy weight on my shoulders of constantly trying to be the perfect mama. No one was putting that weight on me except myself. I felt I didn't deserve to be hurting because I had something I had prayed and yearned for for many years waiting at home for me. I felt that all of these things that made me feel empty would disappear when I had a baby. I hurt even more deeply because that didn't happen. It wasn't my child's responsibility to take years of hurt away from me. I was trying to place such a heavy job on such a sweet little soul. Having a baby filled a void, but it didn't heal me. The only person who could truly walk me through 100 percent healing was my heavenly father.

I think sometimes we believe that after years of struggling with infertility, as soon as the baby is here, it washes away. Don't get me wrong, it does help, but once you let yourself walk through full healing and into full freedom, it's such a beautiful journey. It will make you better in every area of your life. Feeling full freedom is life changing.

After prayer, I went back to my seat and got out my notebook and pen to start processing what I was feeling and what God was speaking to me. Here's part of what I wrote:

Lord, today I choose to let go of all pain and offense I've been carrying from my years of infertility. I choose to healthily grieve, let go and give it to you. The pain was not your plan for me. The disappointment was not your plan for me.

I thank you Lord that I leave lighter than I was when I walked into this conference. I uproot every lie that has been spoken over me and the ones I have believed myself. I rip them out at the root where they can no longer grow. They have no room in my life.

I thank you that whatever you have planned for my future is good. I thank you that all sickness or disease is going to leave mine and my husband's body so we can walk in complete healing. We are made whole in you. You are so, so good!

For the Lord is always good and ready to receive you.
He's so loving that it will amaze you-
so kind that it will astound you!

And he is famous for his faithfulness toward all.

Everyone knows our God can be trusted, for he keeps his promises to every generation!

Psalm 100:5, The Passion Translation

Friends, here are a few questions I want to ask you today:

1. What disappointment have you held on to that you need to let go of and be free from?
2. What do you need to fully grieve in your life?
3. What is a lie you are believing over your life that you need to uproot today?
4. Are you letting the unbelief of others attach itself to you?

5. Are you placing your freedom in some-
    one else's hands or in the Lord's hands
    where it belongs?

6. Are you living your life fully free?

Don't just pull the weed out—rip it out all the
way at the root where it can no longer have a
place in your life.

13

Changed for Good

Infertility changed me. It changed me as a person, wife, mama, friend, Christian, daughter and every other role I fill in life. I have grown stronger. I know I'm capable of anything I put my mind to. Infertility made me a warrior because I kept fighting for what I wanted. No matter what obstacles came my way, I kept fighting.

As a wife, I have grown stronger. Infertility can either push you closer to your spouse or tear you apart. One thing I feel is so important in this journey is ensuring you and your spouse are on the same page. In moments where one of us was ahead, we had to be willing to wait for the other. That was hard at times, but at the end of all of this, we needed to be standing together. We needed to be a united front to prepare our hearts to become parents without bitterness. Our four-and-a-half-year struggle bonded us more than ever. We chose to pursue each other, even on emotionally hard days, and we chose to always keep Christ at the center of our marriage. We chose to meet each other where we were at and lean in—lean into the comfort of the Father and lean into each other. We learned to hold on tighter and not let go.

As a mama, I have grown stronger. It has made me savor every moment with my little love. I've babied him more than I should, held him for far too many naps and only let family watch him, but every time I see that sweet little face, I'm reminded of where I came from, what I fought for and what my responsibility is now. I want to be the absolute best I can be for him. I want to teach him so many things, but most of all to love the Lord with all his heart and that miracles are still real and tangible.

As a daughter, I have grown stronger. I look at my parents and see the encouragers I needed in our hardest times. I see the sacrifices they made and the love they continued to give. I see some of my biggest cheerleaders in life. In hard times, they taught me to look for the light at the end of the tunnel and never stop trying until I reach the end. I see their strength and years of prayer. I see their answered prayers when I see the undeniable joy they have as grandparents.

My in-laws have shown me what true support is and what true prayer warriors are.

They are the definition of people who would do absolutely anything for you to achieve your dreams. They have shown me what it's like to take a child on as their own, how to be fierce encouragers and how to be the absolute best grandparents.

As a friend, I have grown stronger. My tribe has shrunk tremendously since I dealt with infertility and now that I am a mama. Some people didn't know how to be my friend during that time, or simply didn't want to be. That's okay. I became even closer with other people. They prayed with me, cried with me, encouraged me and celebrated with me. I had to choose to know the people that truly loved me would stick by my side. Some of them would wade through the trenches to come take me by the hand and help me out. Everyone goes through hard times. It's the ones who stick it out with you, see you through and cheer you on along the way that are your true friends.

As a Christian, I have grown stronger. Where do I even begin with this one? Every single day I see my son, I'm reminded of the goodness of God! I'm reminded that my prayers were answered, and my promise was fulfilled. I'm reminded that our God is a God of miracles. He's a God that doesn't look at percentages or a diagnosis. He is in the miracle making business. At the end of the day, no matter how tough it was, I chose and declared that He was good! He proved that time and time again to me.

Infertility changes you. I believe you choose whether it changes you in a good or bad way. The things you endure build you up or tear you down. It doesn't mean those hard days won't come. It doesn't mean it's not okay to hurt or be upset. It just means you look at

135

life a little differently. You savor moments more. You find joy in the small things. You continually see how good God is, and how He never leaves you!

14

No Wrong Answer

The questions I get asked the most
these days are ones like these: When are you
having another one? Will you go through IVF
again? Do you want more kids? Are you going
to try for a little girl? Here's the tough part, I
truly don't know the answer to any of those
questions. At the time many were asking us
those questions, we hadn't decided if we
wanted more kids or if we wanted to go
through IVF again. I felt such a weight to make

a decision, knowing what each of these answers would mean for our life.

I had an amazing friend say something to me at a retreat in April of 2019 that completely shifted my perspective. I asked for prayer in our small group for this very thing. I was having a hard time sorting through what I was feeling, and we needed clarity and direction. She said if you were standing before God and your family could look any way you wanted it to, what would that look like? I told her I truly didn't know. That was hard for me to say. Here's what stuck out to me. She said, that's okay. There is no wrong answer.

THERE IS NO WRONG ANSWER.

I felt the weight of my decision because I felt afraid I would make the wrong decision or give the wrong answer. That was a big light-bulb moment for me. Although it was such a simple statement, it was very profound. It made me dig down deep to find out what my feelings truly were.

I no longer feel pressured by the things people say or how having an only child could rob my child of memories and opportunities. Here's the thing—my picture or my husband's picture of what our family should look like is just that—ours. Not theirs. Not yours. So many times, we put pressure on ourselves to look a certain way or live up to certain people's expectations. That's something I decided I'm no longer willing to do. My peace and clarity come from within and from the Lord, not from others.

We continue to live our life to the fullest and savor every adventure and minute together. We open up our hearts and ears and listen. We lean in. We choose to know we have the best author on our side. By doing all these things, we are pretty solidified on our answer now. Does that mean we stop listening to His promptings about this? Absolutely not! We keep listening. We keep leaning in.

One thing we do know for sure is the Lord is not releasing us to pursue fertility treatments again. You know what that would look like for us. We don't have any other frozen embryos. Of what was implanted, one took, the other one didn't and the other five embabies are in heaven waiting to be reunited with their daddy, mama and brother when that day comes. I often wonder what they would have grown to look like and be like. I wonder if any of them are running around heaven, dancing with red hair just like their mama. I wonder if one of the little girls loves to dance just like I did. I dreamed of the day I would take my daughter to her first ballet class, but she has the best dance teacher of all teaching her to dance. I get visions of them in my head, most of them a beautiful redheaded little girl with curly hair, blue eyes and the most infectious smile. I just know that is exactly who Lincoln's twin sister would have been.

This year I got to honor these precious lives at the Moms in the Making conference by hanging their names on a remembrance tree. The year before, I skipped doing this because I believed the lie that those weren't really babies. In my heart, I knew those were my babies. The Lord showed me the deep hurt I carried because I hadn't grieved the loss of what I thought my family would be one day. Those little lives mattered. Those were our future babies and Lincoln's future siblings. Now they have the best Father watching over them.

One day I was sitting in the parking lot at Moms Morning Out staring into a beautiful wooded area. I asked the Lord to speak to me in that moment about what our future family looked like. I wanted to take a deep look and ask myself if the reason I didn't want to expand my family was because of unbelief. I had an overwhelming peace and the Lord told me it was okay. It was okay if I felt my family was complete. He wanted to make sure this is how I truly felt in my heart of hearts. We had a back and forth conversation I desperately needed, and I knew my heart was at peace after that. Let's stop letting others write our story for us. There's only one person I want to be the author of my story. His stories are much more beautiful than anyone else's stories. Who is writing your story?

15

Love Your Mama

As I sit here in your nursery, listening to the rain outside and watching the rise and fall of your chest, I can't help but sit here and hold you a little longer, rock you a little more, studying all your sweet little features. I can't stop staring at your sweet little lips and your beautiful long eyelashes that would rival mine any day. Before you were ever here, I used to sit in this same place and rock in this same chair, dreaming of the day instead of my journal and pen steadily moving in here, I would spend the time with you.

Now I sit here reading the letter I wrote you before you started growing in my belly. Before you even became the little embryo that could. I vividly remember the Lord speaking to me and telling me to write a letter to my future baby. I put it off, not knowing if I could emotionally handle something like this at that time. A few days later, on a Sunday morning at church, one of the sweetest, most encouraging women came up to me and said, I saw this, immediately thought of you, and had to buy it for you. It was a small book called letters to my baby. It had different pages that you write different letters to your baby to commemorate special times in their life. This gift was so special to me, and obviously the Lord was showing me even more that this was something I needed to do. That day I went home, wrote the letter and had such a special prayer time. At the end of the letter I wrote, I can't wait for the day I get to hold you, my sweet miracle baby, Lincoln McCawley Lee, in my arms. I love you already. Love, your Mama. I could feel the Lord's peace washing over me. Now I sit here, and my miracle is in my arms, giving me hugs and kisses, and calling me mama. Those are some of the most special moments that fill my day!

I am praying for you today, friend. Praying you get to experience those same moments. Praying you get that baby or babies that will make you a mama or daddy. I'm praying against all the things that come against you to keep you away from your promise. I'm praying against the fear that tries to fall over you. I'm praying and speaking life into your womb. I'm praying for your finances during this journey. I'm praying for the adoption process you may be going through. I'm praying that all the things that need to come into alignment with you or your spouse's body would. I'm praying you continue to have the strength to push through as you finish your injections or treatments. I'm praying for your heart as you take a break. I'm praying and believing for healing from the top of your head to the soles of your feet. I'm praying for strength for you and your spouse. I'm praying for peace. I'm praying you don't lose hope.

I pray wherever you are in your journey, you take this moment to remind yourself of the promise God has for you! Don't stop praying. You could be on the brink of your miracle!

Epilogue
IVF from the Passenger-Seat
By Bryant Lee

Before bringing you along on our journey through IVF from the passenger's seat, I
want to say thank you to my wife for her brav-
ery in sharing what she had to go through to
see our desires come to pass. We wouldn't
have made it without the support of family and
friends during the journey.

I won't forget when we decided to start
this whole process. I was very reluctant at first
because I heard how expensive it was, and I
really didn't think we had exhausted every

avenue possible before embarking on IVF. At that point, it had been a while and we were not seeing results, so I went with my wife's notion to visit a specialist. We went for the initial consultation and had testing done a few months later. It was a day or two before we got the results back and that was a little nerve-racking, but at the same time, we thought there was probably something simple that could be done to fix the issue. It was the second day after testing, and Angela called with the results. I was anticipating there would be some medicine we would need along with changes in our eating and we should see results in no time. However, it wasn't quite that simple. He told us we had a 1% chance of having a natural born child given our circumstances. I'll never forget where I was at in that moment. A rush of emotions came barreling in while Angela explained what the doctor said. It was only by the grace of

God I didn't hit anyone while driving on Hefner Parkway! I can't speak for everyone who has gone through similar experiences, but I had a wide range of emotions. I would love to tell you I came to my wife's side like a knight in shining armor, but it was more like wondering how I get off this wooden roller coaster I didn't pay to get on! On top of it all, I was heading to an appointment where the couple was going to make their first major purchase as a family. I had to hold it together for me and them for two completely different reasons! After the rush of emotions, Angela and I talked about it that night and took time to pray for a couple of days on what should we do next. Ultimately, we decided to go with IVF.

There was the common hurdle many face in this situation and that was, how are we going to pay for this?? I immediately thought I would just produce enough to cover the cost by putting in extra work. The more I thought about it, the more I was overwhelmed by the thought of producing enough above our cost of living to cover all the medical expenses. That was like taking on the challenge of paying, in full, for a small car in a few short months! There were moments I was driving around saying, Lord, I can't do this on my own. As always, He knows just where we are at.

A week or so went by before we were scheduled for our next appointment, the orientation. I had been working extra time with the hopes of paying for the treatment before the deadline, not realizing God had already orchestrated everything for us. The day we were scheduled to go for our initial appointment to begin the process, I met with someone in hopes of creating more business. I went in and told them about our situation. They are people we trust and knew they supported us, so we felt comfortable sharing our story with them. After going through the whole situation with them, I was expecting a response of yes, I'll send more clients your way and we'll pray for you. They asked some pointed questions about the process and I ended up telling them it was a money issue. They said, come with me. Obviously I did, without knowing what in the world was going on! What happened next is something I'll never forget.

They asked, how much is it? I proceeded to tell them the amount while thinking—is this really happening!?! They told their assistant to write a check to cover the amount we needed! There wasn't a dry eye in the room. They said they've been praying about it before I came to them and felt like they were supposed to do it. I could barely breathe at this point. I couldn't wait to tell Angela when I met her at the appointment, but I knew if I told her while I was driving, we would put others in danger! All I told her was I had something to show her before we went in. If you know Angela, you know suspense drives her crazy!

We met at the doctor's office, and I pulled the check out to show her. She held it in shock! I'll never forget the look on her face. I think I remember her asking, is this real?! It was an amazing moment. When I look back on everything that happened up to that point, I saw it as an Abraham and Isaac moment. God knew as Abraham and Isaac were going up the mountain, there would be a ram in the thicket. Ram's horns are designed to avoid getting caught in thickets, so you know it was an uncommon moment where God met them at their point of obedience. Abraham and Isaac didn't know the ram was coming up the other side of the mountain to meet them, just like we didn't know God was bringing our ram up the side of our mountain. All we knew was that we had to obey.

We began the process with the financial hurdle crossed off, but we knew it was just the beginning. We heard all the stories and statistics about people going through IVF for the first time. Have you ever noticed that when you begin something it seems like all the negative people show up to tell you why something may not happen? Or when they knew someone (cousin, sister, aunt or friend they haven't seen since high school) that went through the same thing and it didn't work out for them? I digress. Day after day, things were nerve-wracking. Through all the ups and downs, we had to remind ourselves of what God had done for us up to that point. I had a very busy schedule with work and she had to come along for the ride most of the time. I had to help Angela with shots in some of the most unconventional places. It wasn't planned that way, but circumstances forced it.

The two weeks after the initial egg retrieval were intense. It was probably the longest two weeks of our life. I would love to say we had it all together most days, but many of them we didn't. With God's grace and the support of family members, we made it through. We had to be careful who we talked to during that time to make sure our faith and mental health stayed intact. When the day came, they called Angela with the results and told her the words she longed to hear for years—you're pregnant.

It really seems like we went from one intense moment to the next. Now we had to go through the process to make sure our baby was going to make it. Just as the process began with some unexpected events, having our child ended with unexpected moments as well.

We ended up having a c-section when we ex-pected Angela to give birth naturally. Let me remind you that Angela doesn't do well with the unknown, so I did what I knew to do—be strong and give her words of encouragement. My biggest concern during the c-section was our doctor's nonchalant attitude. It was like business as usual for her and her assistants. They were laughing and having a good time. I needed them at a level ten emotionally be-cause that's where we were, not knowing we were her fourth procedure of the night! Everything we endured was worth it the mo-ment a healthy baby boy was placed into my arms for the first time!

But those who trust in the
LORD will find new strength.
They will soar high on wings
like eagles.
They will run and not grow
weary.
They will walk and not faint.
Isaiah 40:31
NLT

Letter from the Author

Thank you for choosing to support me and come along on this journey by reading my book. I've always dreamed of becoming a published author, and so many of you supported me and made this possible. Life has changed so much since I started writing. The little baby I wrote about is now a full blown, non-stop talking three-year-old. He is so full of adventure, joy and humor, and he loves so hard. He loves all things outdoors and adores music, or "Praise you Jesus" music as he calls it, and riding his new bike with training wheels. He continually teaches me so much and makes me want to be a better person.

I have connected with the most beautiful community of infertility warriors. I am honored and humbled to do life and ministry with them. Seeing so many miracles happen over and over again makes me continually pray, do it again, Lord! Do it again!

I would love to connect more with you! If you are seeking community or need prayer please reach out to me at whileinwaiting@yahoo.com or on Instagram @while_in_waiting. You can also continue to follow our journey on my blog at www.whileinwaiting.com.

Acknowledgements

To My Number One Bryant,

I am incredibly blessed to call you my husband and be on this adventure of life together. If I had my choice of anyone in the world, I would choose you over and over again. I know I've told you this before, but thank you. Thank you for joining me hand in hand through this journey of life, navigating infertility with me and never leaving my side. If anything, you only pulled me in closer. You are supportive, encouraging, smart, kindhearted, strong, so funny and just the best husband and daddy to our little boy. Seeing you become a dad made me fall even more in love with you and see you in a whole new way. I love you to the moon and back.

To My Little Linc,

You gave me the greatest gift in life by making me a mama. You are truly my miracle boy. You may be small, but you teach me things on a daily basis. You love hard, laugh all the time, love to talk about Jesus, and you have the best imagination. Thank you for the gift you are to me. I can't wait to see you grow and walk in all the amazing things God has in store for you!

To My Parents,
Grammy and Pop Pop:
Thank you! You have always been my biggest cheerleaders in life. I can't imagine having better parents than the both of you. Thank you for believing in me, pulling me through so many tough times, speaking truth and sharing wisdom. I have learned so much by watching y'all lead by example. You taught me how to parent

well one day and now as I'm walking in that, I get to see you flourish as grandparents. A dream come true for both of us.

To the Lee Family,

Poppy and GoGo: From day one, you treated me as your own. I am forever thankful for how incredibly loving, welcoming and supportive you are. Your constant laughter always makes me feel right at home.

Faith and Mase: I gained an incredible little brother and sister when I became a Lee, and it has been so fun getting to experience younger siblings. Seeing how much my son adores his aunt and uncle is so special to me.

To the Tisdale's,

Mimi and Papa: Thank you for your strength and leadership to help us see our dreams become a reality. You continually challenge us to be everything that God calls us to be. Seeing you as grandparents is such a joy!

To My Brother,

I hate to admit it, but over time, you have become one of my very best friends. From helping chase people bothering me on the playground in elementary school to me forcing you to hold your nephew for the first time, you have always been there for me. Thank you for the daily laughs. I love all of our talks and how we have grown so close.

To My Sisters,

You two have not only become my biggest cheerleaders in getting this book finished and in life, but you two have also become my best friends. I love both of you and your children beyond words. Life brought us together, and the Lord has knit the most amazing sisterhood and accountability group I could have ever asked for. I love you both so much!

To My Grandparents,
Not all of you are with us now, but you have always been an inspiration to me. You have brought a life full of fun, songs, shopping trips, dinners, family gatherings and a lifetime of memories. I love you all so much.

To Our Family,
The list would be forever long if I named all of you individually, but know we are thankful for each and every one of you. Your prayers and support have meant the world to Bryant and me. We are thankful to do life with such a strong support system.

To Whitney,

You have showed up day after day holding me accountable, listening to me talk through what needed to go on these pages, encouraging me to not give up, praying for me, and reminding me of all my deadlines I needed to meet. You have been a God send through this whole process and I couldn't have made it through without you helping push me along. I'm so thankful to call you my forever friend!

To My Moms in the Making Family,

I am forever changed by you! You all have been such an amazing community, support system, prayer warriors, leaders, and the best friends a girl could ask for. Thank you for helping me realize areas I needed to change and grow,

helping me walk through healing and helping
me fall even more in love with Jesus.

To the Zellner Family,
You saw me through the thick of my journey
and loved me through all of it. Your kids
helped bring me so much joy during one of the
hardest times in my life.
Tara, thank you for taking time every day to
stop working, share words of wisdom and be
my confidant through all of this. I'm forever
thankful for you.
Grant, thanks for always making me laugh!
Now go eat some cheese. Lynzee, Creede, and
Cayden, I will always cherish you three. Wawa
loves you! You will always be family to me.

To the Levinsons,

We can never say thank you enough! You both lead incredibly well and create an amazing team in a family environment. We always felt at home and ourselves with y'all. Thank you for believing in my husband and challenging him to be the best he could be. The growth he experienced with y'all is immeasurable. I saw a change in him he needed, and I know you helped pull that out of him. We love you!

To My Friends,

To list everyone who helped me individually would take up at least ten more pages. I'm immensely grateful for those of you who stuck it out with me through the hard times, prayed for me, opened your homes and made them a safe place, and for all the encouragement you each shared with me. I'm one lucky girl to have the

absolute best friends. Thank you for being
you! I love you!

To my amazing editor Emily and designer Alexis,
I could never thank the both of you enough
for all of your hard work. Thank you for stick-
ing with me and being a vital part of this book
becoming a reality for me. You were both absolutely amazing to work with and I hope we
get to work together again in the future.

Lastly, But Most Importantly, To My Loving
Savior,
You gave me nudge after nudge to begin writing by starting my blog and then leading me
here. Walking hand in hand with you through
my fertility journey and writing this book
stretched me in ways I didn't know were possible. I have learned so much as you have paint-

ed the most beautiful pictures and helped me know what words were meant to be shared. I will never stop being amazed by you.

Made in the USA
Coppell, TX
31 October 2020

40543907R10100

Did you know that 6.1 million women face infertility in America? Despite that shocking statistic, many women feel alone in their struggle to conceive. Angela was one of those women. She felt alone and ashamed in her struggle with infertility until God provided miracle after miracle for her family and an incredible community of infertility warriors that have carried her through.

In her story of heartbreak and hope, Angela shares her journey with infertility, IVF, and the birth of her beautiful baby boy to encourage other women who struggle with infertility. Through her honesty, humor and encouragement, you are sure to be inspired by Angela's journey and filled with renewed hope for the battles you are facing.

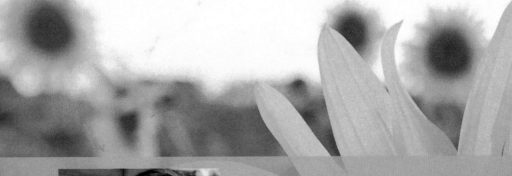

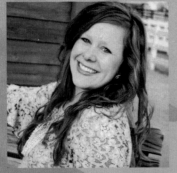

Angela Lee writes at www.whileinwaiting.com as an encourager and advocate for the fertility community. Her goal is to spread hope and help others keep their eyes fixed on Jesus while they are in their waiting season. She is an Oklahoma born and raised girl that now resides in South Carolina with her sweet, southern husband, Bryant, and her wild, adventurous son, Lincoln.

To keep up with Angela and her family, you can follow her @while_in_waiting on Instagram.

ISBN 9780578761022

90000

9 780578 761022